CW00486788

KETO DIET FOR WOMEN

The Ultimate and Complete Guide to Lose Weight Quickly, Regain Confidence, and Balance Hormones at The Same Time

By Melissa Cook

This document is geared towards providing exact and reliable information in regards to the topic and issue covered. The publication is sold with the idea that the publisher is not required to render accounting, officially permitted, or otherwise, qualified services. If advice is necessary, legal or professional, a practiced individual in the profession should be ordered.

- From a declaration of principles which was accepted and approved equally by a committee of the American bar association and a committee of publishers and associations.

The information herein is offered for informational purposes solely and is universal as such. The presentation of the information is without a contract or any type of guarantee assurance.

The trademarks used are without any consent, and the publication of the trademark is without permission or backing by the trademark owner. All trademarks and brands within this book are for clarifying purposes only and are owned by the owners themselves, not affiliated with this document.

Contents

Introduction

The keto diet is a diet that has higher and lower fat values. It decreases glucose & insulin levels and changes the body's digestion away from carbohydrates and more towards fat & ketones. A word used in a low-carb diet is "Ketogenic." The concept is to provide more calories from fat and protein and few from sugars. The consumption of a high, low-sugar diet, adequate-protein, is used in medicine to achieve difficult (unstable) epilepsy control in young people. Instead of sugar, the diet allows the body to eat fats. Usually, the nutritious starches are converted to sugar, which will then be distributed throughout the body and is particularly important in filling the mind's work. Keto diet can cause enormous declines in the levels of glucose and insulin.

How food affects your body

Our metabolic procedures survive if we do not get the right details, and our well-being declines. We can get overweight, malnourished, and at risk for the worsening of diseases and disorders, such as inflammatory disease, diabetes, and cardiovascular disease if women get an unhealthy amount of essential nutrients or nourishment that provides their body with inadequate guidance. The dietary supplements allow the cells in our bodies to serve their essential capacities. This quote from a well-known workbook shows how dietary supplements are important for our physical work. Supplements are the nourishment feed substances necessary for the growth, development, and support of the body's capacities. Fundamental claimed that when a supplement is absent, capability sections and thus decrease in human health. The metabolic processes are delayed when the intake of supplements usually may not fulfill the cell activity's supplement requirements.

The keto diet involves keeping to a relatively low-carb, high-fat diet to put the body into a physiological state called ketosis. This makes fat intake increasingly productive for the health. When starting the diet, the ketogenic diet can induce a decrease in the drive, as the dieter will suffer side effects of carb removal and possibly low carb influenza. Whenever the detox and influenza-like symptoms have gone, and the dieter has transitioned to the reduced way of living, leading to weight loss from the diet, the charisma would in all likelihood reset and probably be comparable to earlier. Although the drive alert has a lot of credibility in the mainstream, in other words, supplementation provides advice to our bodies on how to function. In this sense, nourishment can be seen as a source of "information for the body." Pondering food along these lines gives one a view of the nourishment beyond calories or grams, fantastic food sources, or bad food sources. Instead of avoiding food sources, this perspective pushes us to reflect on the nutrients we can add. Instead of reviewing nourishment as the enemy, we look at nourishment to reduce health and disease by having the body look after ability.

Kidney and Heart Disease

When the body is low in electrolytes and fluid over the increased pee, electrolyte loss, such as magnesium, sodium, and potassium, can be caused. This will render people inclined to suffer serious kidney problems. Flushing out is not a joke and can lead to light-headedness, damage to the kidney, or kidney problems. Just like electrolytes are essential for the heart's standard stomping, this can place a dieter at the risk of cardiac arrhythmia. "Electrolyte appears to lack are not joking, and that may bring in an irregular heartbeat, that can be harmful,"

Yo-yo Dieting designs

When individuals encounter difficulties staying on the prohibitive diet indefinitely, the keto diet will also cause yo-yo dieting. That can have other adverse effects on the body.

Other effects

Other responses can involve terrible breath, fatigue, obstruction, irregular menstrual periods, reduced bone density, and trouble with rest. For even the most part, other consequences are not so much considered since it is impossible to observe dieters on a long-term assumption to discover the food schedule's permanent effects.

Wholesome Concerns

"There is still a dread amongst healthcare professionals that certain high intakes of extremely unhealthy fats will have a longer journey negative effect," she explained. Weight loss will also, for the time being, complicate the data. As overweight people get in form, paying less attention to how they do so, they sometimes end up with much better lipid profiles and blood glucose levels.

In comparison, the keto diet is extremely low in particular natural ingredients, fruits, nuts, and veggies that are as nutritious as a whole. Without these supplements, fiber, some carbohydrates, minerals, including phytochemicals that come along with these nourishments, will move through people on a diet. In the long run, this has vital public health consequences, such as bone degradation and increased risk of infinite diseases.

Sodium

The mixture of sodium (salt), fat, sugar, including bunches of sodium, will make inexpensive food more delicious for many people. However, diets rich in sodium will trigger fluid retention, which is why you can feel puffy, bloated, or swelled up in the aftermath of consuming cheap food. For those with pulse problems, a diet rich in sodium is also harmful. Sodium can increase circulatory stress and add weight to the cardiovascular structure. If one survey reveals, about % of grown-ups lose how much salt is in their affordable food meals. The study looked at 993 adults and found that the initial prediction was often smaller than the actual figure (1,292 mg). This suggests the sodium gauges in the abundance of 1,000 mg is off. One affordable meal could be worth a significant proportion of your day.

Impact on the Respiratory Framework

An overabundance of calories can contribute to weight gain from cheap foods. This will add to the weight. Obesity creates the risk of respiratory conditions, including asthma with shortness of breath. The extra pounds can put pressure on the heart and lungs, and with little intervention, side effects can occur. When you walk, climb stairs, or work out, you can notice trouble breathing. For youngsters, the possibility of respiratory problems is especially obvious. One research showed that young people who consume cheap food at least three days a week are bound to develop asthma.

Impact on the focal sensory system

For the time being, cheap food may satisfy hunger; however, long-haul effects are more detrimental. Individuals who consume inexpensive food and processed bakery items are 51 percent bound to generate depression than people who do not eat or eat either of those foods.

Impact on the conceptive framework

The fixings in cheap food and lousy nourishment can affect your money. One analysis showed that phthalates are present in prepared nourishment. Phthalates are synthetic compounds that can mess with the way your body's hormones function. Introduction to substantial amounts of these synthetics, like birth absconds, could prompt regenerative problems.

Impact on the integumentary framework (skin, hair, nails)

The food you eat may affect your skin's appearance, but it's not going to be the food you imagine. The responsibility for skin dry out breakouts has traditionally been claimed by sweets and sticky nourishments such as pizza. Nevertheless, as per the Mayo Clinic, there are starches. Carb-rich foods cause glucose jumps, and these sudden leaps in glucose levels can induce inflammation of the skin. Additionally, as shown by one investigation, young people and young women who consume inexpensive food at any pace three days a week are expected to create skin inflammation. Dermatitis is a skin disease that causes dry, irritated skin spots that are exacerbated.

Impact on the skeletal framework (bones)

Acids in the mouth can be enlarged by carbohydrates and sugar in inexpensive food and treated food. These acids may distinguish tooth lacquer. Microorganisms can take hold when the tooth veneer disappears, and depressions can occur. Weight will also prompt issues with bone thickness and bulk. The more severe chance of falling and breaking bones is for heavy individuals. It is important to continue training, develop muscles that support the bones, and sustain a balanced diet to prevent bone loss. One investigation showed that the measure of calories, sugar, and sodium in cheap food meals remains, to a large degree, constant because of attempts to bring problems to light and make women more intelligent consumers. As women get busier and eat out more often, it could have antagonistic effects on women and America's healthcare structure.

Chapter 1: Keto Diet and Its Benefits

In the case of a ketogenic diet, the aim is to restrict carbohydrate intake to break down fat for power. When this occurs, to produce ketones that are by-products of the metabolism, the liver breaks down fat. These ketones are used in the absence of glucose to heat the body. A ketogenic diet takes the body into a "ketosis" mode. A metabolic condition that happens as ketone bodies in the blood contains most of the body's energy rather than glucose from carbohydrate-produced foods (such as grains, all sources of sugar or fruit). This compares with a glycolytic disorder, where blood glucose produces most of the body's power.

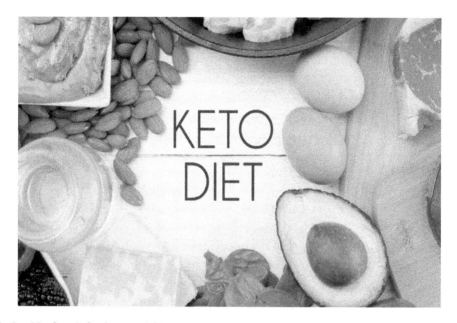

1.1. Keto Diet and its Success

The keto diet is successful in many studies, especially among obese men and women. The results suggest that KD can help manage situations such as:

- Obesity.

- Heart disease.

It is difficult to relate the ketogenic diet to cardiovascular disease risk factors. Several studies have shown that keto diets may contribute to substantial reductions in overall cholesterol, rises in levels of HDL cholesterol, decreases in levels of triglycerides and decreases in levels of LDL cholesterol, as well as possible changes in levels of blood pressure.

- Neurological disorders, including Alzheimer's, dementia, multiple sclerosis and Parkinson's.

- Polycystic ovarian syndrome (PCOS), among women of reproductive age, is the most prevalent endocrine condition.
- Certain forms of cancer, including cancers of the liver, colon, pancreas and ovaries.
- Diabetes Type 2. Among type 2 diabetics, it can also minimize the need for drugs.
- Seizure symptoms and seizures.
- And others.

1.2. Why Do the Ketogenic Diet

By exhausting the body from its sugar store, Ketogenic works to start sorting fat and protein for vitality, inducing ketosis (and weight loss).

1. Helps in weight loss

To convert fat into vitality, it takes more effort than it takes to turn carbohydrates into vitality. A ketogenic diet along these lines can help speed up weight loss. In comparison, because the diet is rich in protein, it doesn't leave you starving as most diets do. Five findings uncovered tremendous weight loss from a ketogenic diet in a meta-examination of 13 complex randomized controlled preliminaries.

2. Diminishes skin break out

There are different causes for the breakout of the skin, and food and glucose can be established. Eating a balanced diet of prepared and refined sugars can alter gut microorganisms and emphasize sensational variances in glucose, both of which would affect the skin's health. Therefore, that is anything but surprising that a keto diet may reduce a few instances of skin inflammation by decreasing carb entry.

3. May help diminish the danger of malignancy

There has been a lot of study on the ketogenic diet and how it could effectively forestall or even cure those malignant growths. One investigation showed that the ketogenic diet might be a corresponding effective treatment with chemotherapy and radiation in people with malignancy. It is because it can cause more oxidative concern than in ordinary cells in malignancy cells.

Some hypotheses indicate that it may decrease insulin entanglements, which could be linked to some cancers because the ketogenic diet lowers elevated glucose.

4. Improves heart health

There is some indication that the diet will boost cardiac health by lowering cholesterol by accessing the ketogenic diet in a balanced manner (which looks at avocados as a healthy fat rather than pork skins). One research showed that LDL ("Terrible") cholesterol levels fundamentally expanded among those adopting the keto diet. In turn, the LDL ("terrible") cholesterol fell.

5. May secure mind working

More study into the ketogenic diet and even the mind is needed. A few studies indicate that the keto diet has Neuro-protective effects. These can help treat or curtail Parkinson's, Alzheimer's, and even some rest problems. One research also showed that young people had increased and psychological work during a ketogenic diet.

6. Possibly lessens seizures

The theory that the combination of fat, protein, and carbohydrates modifies how vitality is utilized by the body, inducing ketosis. Ketosis is an abnormal level of Ketone in the blood. In people with epilepsy, ketosis will prompt a reduction in seizures.

7. Improves health in women with PCOS

An endocrine condition that induces augmented ovaries with pimples is polycystic ovarian disorder PCOS). On the opposite, a high-sugar diet can affect those with PCOS. On the ketogenic diet and PCOS, there are not many clinical tests. One pilot study involving five women on 24 weeks showed that the ketogenic diet:

- Aided hormone balance
- Improved luteinizing hormone (ILH)/follicle-invigorating hormone (FSH) proportions
- Increased weight loss
- Improved fasting insulin

For children who suffer the adverse effects of a particular problem (such as Lennox-gastaut disease or Rett disorder) and do not respond to seizure prescription, keto is also prescribed as suggested by the epilepsy foundation.

They note that the number of seizures these children had can be greatly reduced by keto, with 10 to 15 percent turns out to be sans seizure. It may also help patients to reduce the portion of their prescription in some circumstances. Be it as it can, the ketogenic diet still many effective trials to back up its advantages. For adults with epilepsy, the keto diet can likewise be helpful. It was considered as preferable to other diets in supporting people with:

- Epilepsy
- Type 2 diabetes
- Type 1 diabetes
- High blood pressure
- Heart disease
- Polycystic ovary syndrome
- Fatty liver disease
- Cancer
- Migraines

- Alzheimer's infection
- Parkinson's infection
- Chronic inflammation
- High blood sugar levels
- Obesity

The ketogenic diet will be beneficial, regardless of whether you are not in danger from any of these disorders. A portion of the advantages that are enjoyed by the vast majority are:

- An increment in vitality
- Improved body arrangement
- Better cerebrum work
- A decline in aggravation

As should be clear, the ketogenic diet has a vast variety of advantages, but is it preferable to other diets?

8. Treating epilepsy — the origins of the ketogenic diet

Until sometime in 1998, the major analysis on epilepsy and the keto diets was not distributed. Of about 150 children, almost each of whom had several seizures a week, despite taking two psychosis drugs in either situation. The children were given a one-year initial ketogenic diet. Around 34 percent of infants, or slightly more than 33 percent, had a 90 percent decline in seizures after three months.

The healthy diet was claimed to be "more feasible than just a substantial lot of new anticonvulsant medications and is much endured by families and kids when it is effective." Not only was the keto diet supportive. It was, however, more useful than other drugs usually used.

9. Improving blood pressure with the ketogenic diet

A low-sugar intake is more effective at reducing the pulse than just a low-fat or moderate-fat diet. Restricting starches often provides preferable results over the mix of a low-fat regimen and a relaxing weight-loss/pulse.

10. The power to improve Alzheimer's disease

Alzheimer's disease patients also agree with organic chemistry." high sugar acceptance deepens academic performance in patient populations with Alzheimer's infectious disease." It means that more starches are consumed in the cerebrum. Will the reverse (trying to eat fewer carbs) improve the functioning of the cerebrum?

Other mental health benefits that ketone bodies have:

- They forestall neuronal loss.
- They ensure synapses against various sorts of damage.
- They save neuron work.

•

1.3. The Benefits of Ketogenic Diet

The board provides many substantial advantages when choosing a ketogenic diet for diabetes. Living in a stable ketosis state causes a tremendous change in blood glucose regulation and weight loss. Other frequent advantages provided include:

- Improvements in insulin affectability
- Lower circulatory strain
- Usually enhancements in cholesterol levels.
- Reduced reliance on taking drugs

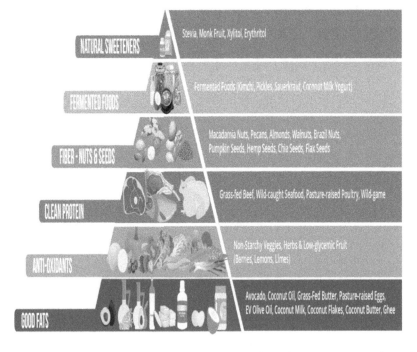

We send you a short science behind the ketogenic diet in this book and how it attempts to give these particular benefits.

1. Weight loss and support

The ketogenic diet's significant benefit is achieving accelerated weight loss, reducing starches necessary to be in a ketosis state, causing both a noteworthy decrease in muscle vs. fats and bulk increase and maintenance. Studies have shown that a low-carb, keto diet can produce an all-inclusive duration of solid weight loss. For one year, a big person had the opportunity to lose, by and large, 15 kilograms. It was 3 kg, which is more than the low-fat food used in the study carried out.

2. Blood glucose control

The other main reason for maintaining a ketogenic diet for people with diabetes is its ability to reduce and regulate glucose levels. The substitute (macronutrient) that improves glucose the most is starch. Since the keto diet is low in starch, the greater rises in glucose are dispensed with. Ketogenic diets prove that they are effective in reducing hba1c, a long-term blood glucose regulation percentage. A natural decrease of 17 mmol/mol (1.5 percent) in hba1c levels for persons with type 2 diabetes. People with other forms of diabetes, such as diabetes and LADA, can also expect to see a strong decline in glucose levels and increase control. Remember that if an increase in blood glucose regulation is sustained over different years, this will reduce intricacies. It is necessary to play it safe for those on insulin, or otherwise at risk of hypos, to avoid the incidence of hypos.

Decreasing drug reliance on diabetes. Since it is so effective at lowering glucose levels, the keto diet provides the added benefit of allowing people with type 2 diabetes to decrease their dependency on diabetes medication.

Persons on insulin and other hypertension prescriptions (Sulphonylureas & Glinides, for example) may need to reduce their portions before initiating a ketogenic diet to avoid hypotension. For advice on this, contact your primary care provider.

3. Insulin affectability

To further restore insulin affectability, a ketogenic diet has emerged since it dispenses with the root driver of insulin obstruction, which is too high insulin levels in the bloodstream. This diet advances supported periods with low insulin since low carbohydrate levels indicate lower insulin levels. A high diet of starch resembles putting petroleum on the insulin obstruction fire. A more influential need for insulin is indicated by elevated sugar, and this aggravates insulin opposition. A ketogenic diet, by correlation, turns down insulin levels since fat is the least insulin-requiring macronutrient. In comparison, bringing the insulin levels down also helps with fat intake, provided that elevated insulin levels inhibit fat breakdown. The body will differentiate fat cells at the point that insulin levels decrease for several hours.

4. Hypertension control

It is estimated that 16 million people in the U.K. suffer from hypertension. Hypertension, for example, cardiovascular disease, stroke, and renal disease, is related to the scope of health disorders. Different studies have demonstrated that a ketogenic diet can reduce circulatory stress levels in overweight or type 2 diabetes people. It is also a part of metabolic imbalance.

5. Cholesterol levels

For the most part, ketogenic diets bring in reductions in cholesterol levels. LDL cholesterol levels are usually reduced, and HDL cholesterol levels increase, which is healthy. The amount of absolute cholesterol to HDL is possibly the most substantiated proportion of safe cholesterol. It can be effectively detected by taking the full cholesterol result and partitioning it by your HDLS result. It indicates good cholesterol, on the off chance that the amount you get is 3.5 or lower. Study findings suggest that ketogenic diets are normally possible to increase this proportion of good cholesterol.

After starting a ketogenic, a few individuals can display an expansion in LDL and all-out cholesterol. It is generally taken as a bad indicator, but this does not speak of compounding in heart health if the absolute cholesterol to HDL ratio is appropriate.

Cholesterol is a confounding topic, and if your cholesterol levels essentially shift on a ketogenic diet, your PCP is the optimization technique of exhortation. More simple mental results. Other typically announced advantages of eating a ketogenic diet are emotional insight, an increased capacity to center, and superior memory. Expanding the admission of omega-3 healthy fats, such as those present in slick fish such as salmon, fish, and mackerel, will boost the state of mind and the ability to read. It is because omega-3 extends an unsaturated fat called DHAS, which makes up 15 to 30 percent of the cerebrum of females. The discovery of beta-hydroxybutyrate, a type of Ketone, allows for long-term memory work to be facilitated.

6. Satiety

The effects of ketogenic diets impact malnutrition. As the body responds to being in a ketosis state, it becomes acclimatized to obtain vitality from muscle to fat ratio differentiation, which will alleviate appetite and desires.

They are possible at:

- **Reducing desires**
- **Reducing inclination for sugary nourishments**
- **Helping you feel full for more**

Weight loss will also reduce leptin levels attributable to a ketogenic diet, which will increase the affectability of leptin and thus gain satiety.

1.4. Keto Shopping List

A keto diet meal schedule for women above 5o+ years and a menu that will transform the body. Generally speaking, the keto diet is low in carbohydrates, high in fat and moderate in protein. While adopting a ketogenic diet, carbs are routinely reduced to under 50 grams every day, but stricter and looser adaptations of the diet exist.

• Proteins can symbolize about 20 percent of strength requirements, whereas carbohydrates are usually restricted to 5 percent.

• The body retains its fat for the body to use as energy production.

Most of the cut carbs should be supplanted by fats and convey about 75% of your all-out caloric intake.

The body processes ketones while it is in ketosis, particles released from cholesterol in the blood glucose is low, as yet another source of energy.

Because fat is always kept a strategic distance from its unhealthy content, research demonstrates that the keto diet is essentially better than low-fat diets to advance weight reduction.

In contrast, keto diets minimize desire and improve satiation, which is especially useful when getting in shape.

Fatty cuts of PROTEIN: *Keto Diet Shopping list*

NUTS AND SEEDS:
1. MACADAMIA NUTS+BUTTER
2. BRAZIL NUTS+BUTTER
3. PECANS+BUTTER
4. WALNUTS
5. PUMPKIN SEEDS
6. ALMONDS +BUTTER

1. GROUND BEEF - RIBEYE STEAK
2. PORK BELLY ROAST +BACON
3. BEEF OR PORK SAUSAGE
4. WILD CAUGHT SALMON
5. SARDINES OR TUNA
6. CHICKEN THIGHS OR LEGS
7. TURKEY LEGS
8. DEER STEAKS
9. EGGS
10. DUCK EGGS
11.

Green Leafy VEGGIES:
1. BROCCOLI
2. CAULIFLOWER
3. GREEN BEANS
4. BRUSSEL SPROUTS
5. KALE
6. SPINACH
7. CHARD
8. CABBAGE
9. BOK CHOY
10. CELERY
11. ARUGULA
12. ASPARAGUS
13. ZUCCHINI
14. YELLOW SQUASH
15. MUSHROOMS
16. OLIVES
17. ARTICHOKE
18. CUCUMBERS
19. ONIONS
20. GARLIC
21. OKRA

FRUITS AND BERRIES:
1. POMEGRANATE
2. GRAPEFRUIT
3. BLUEBERRIES
4. RASPBERRIES
5. LEMON
6. LIME
7. AVOCADO

FATS:
1. BUTTER
2. OLIVE OIL
3. COCONUT OIL
4. COCONUT BUTTER
5. MCT OIL
6. AVOCADO
7. GHEE
8. BACON GREASE
9. AVOCADO OIL

MUST HAVE MISCELLANEOUS:
1. ALMOND+COCONUT FLOUR
2. COCONUT BUTTER
3. 85% DARK CHOCOLATE
4. PORK RINDS
5. COCONUT CREAM
6. COCONUT FLAKES

1.5. Keto-Friendly Foods to Eat

Meals and bites should be based on the accompanying nourishment when following a ketogenic diet:

Eggs: pastured eggs are the best choice for all-natural eggs.

Meat: hamburger grass- nourished, venison, pork, organ meat, and buffalo.

Full-fat dairy: yogurt, cream and margarine.

Full-fat Cheddar: Cheddar, mozzarella, brie, cheddar goat and cheddar cream.

Nuts and seeds: almonds, pecans, macadamia nuts, peanuts, pumpkin seeds, and flaxseeds.

Poultry: turkey and chicken.

Fatty fish: Wild-got salmon, herring, and mackerel

Nut margarine: Natural nut, almond, and cashew spreads.

Vegetables that are not boring: greens, broccoli, onions, mushrooms, and peppers.

Condiments: salt, pepper, lemon juice, vinegar, flavors and crisp herbs.

Fats: coconut oil, olive oil, coconut margarine, avocado oil, and sesame oil.

Avocados: it is possible to add whole avocados to practically any feast or bite.

1.6. Nourishments to avoid

Although adopting a keto diet, keep away from carbohydrate-rich nutrients.

It is important to restrict the accompanying nourishments:

- **Sweetened beverages:** beer, juice, better teas, and drinks for sports.
- **Pasta:** noodles and spaghetti.
- **Grains and vegetable articles:** maize, rice, peas, oats for breakfast
- **Starchy vegetables:** Butternut squash, Potatoes, beans, sweet potatoes, pumpkin and peas.
- **Beans and vegetables:** chickpeas, black beans, kidney beans and lentils.
- **Fruit:** citrus, apples, pineapple and bananas.
- **Sauces containing high-carbohydrates:** BBQ' sauce, a sugar dressing with mixed greens, and dipping's.
- **Hot and bread items:** white bread, whole wheat bread, wafers, cookies, doughnuts, rolls, etc.
- **Sweets and sweet foods:** honey, ice milk, candy, chocolate syrup, agave syrup, coconut sugar.
- **Blended refreshments:** Sugar-blended cocktails and beer.

About the assumption that carbs should be small, low-glycemic organic goods, for example, when a keto-macronutrient is served, spread, berries may be satisfied with restricted quantities. Be sure to choose safe sources of protein and eliminate prepared sources of food and bad fats.

It is worth keeping the accompanying stuff away from:

28

1. Diet nutrients: Foods containing counterfeit hues, contaminants and carbohydrates, such as aspartame and sugar alcohols.

2. Unhealthy fats: Such as corn and canola oil, include shortening, margarine, and cooking oils.

3. Processed foods: Fast foods, bundled food sources, and frozen meats, such as wieners and meats for lunch.

1.8. One week Keto Diet Plan

(Day 1): Monday

Breakfast: Eggs fried in seasoned butter served over vegetables.

Lunch: A burger of grass-bolstered with avocado, mushrooms, and cheddar on a tray of vegetables.

Dinner: Pork chops and French beans sautéed in vegetable oil.

(Day 2): Tuesday

Breakfast: Omelet of mushroom.

Lunch: Salmon, blended vegetables, tomato, and celery on greens.

Dinner: Roast chicken and sautéed cauliflower.

(Day 3): Wednesday

Breakfast: Cheddar cheese, eggs, and bell peppers.

Lunch: Blended veggies with hard-bubbled eggs, avocado, turkey, and cheddar.

Dinner: Fried salmon sautéed in coconut oil.

(Day 4): Thursday

Breakfast: Granola with bested full-fat yogurt.

Lunch: Steak bowl of cheddar, cauliflower rice, basil, avocado, as well as salsa.

Dinner: Bison steak and mushy cauliflower.

(Day 5): Friday

Breakfast: Pontoons of Avocado egg (baked).

Lunch: Chicken served with Caesar salad.

Dinner: Pork, with veggies.

(Day 6): Saturday

Breakfast: Avocado and cheddar with cauliflower.

Lunch: Bunless burgers of salmon.

Dinner: Parmesan cheddar with noodles topped with meatballs.

(Day 7): Sunday

Breakfast: Almond Milk, pecans and Chia pudding.

Lunch: Cobb salad made of vegetables, hard-boiled eggs, mango, cheddar, and turkey.

Dinner: Curry chicken.

Chapter 2: Health Concerns for Women Over 50+

This chapter will give you a detailed view of the health concerns for women over 50.

2.1. Menopause

Healthy maturation includes large propensities such as eating healthy, avoiding regular prescription mistakes, monitoring health conditions, receiving suggested screenings, or being dynamic. Getting more seasoned involves change, both negative and positive, but you can admire maturing on the off chance of understanding your body's new things and finding a way to maintain your health. As you age, a wide range of things happens to your body. Unexpectedly, your skin, bones, and even cerebrum may start to carry on. Try not to let the advances that accompany adulthood get you off guard.

Here's a segment of the normal ones:

1. The Bones: In mature age, bones may become slender and progressively weaker, especially in women, leading to the delicate bone disease known as osteoporosis once in a while. Diminishing bones and decreasing bone mass can put you at risk for falls that can occur in broken bones without much of a stretch result. Make sure you talk to your doctor about what you can do to prevent falls and osteoporosis.

2. The Heart: While a healthy diet and normal exercise can keep your heart healthy, it may turn out to be somewhat amplified, lowering your pulse and thickening the heart dividers.

3. The Sensory system and Mind: It can trigger changes in your reflexes and even your skills by becoming more seasoned. While dementia is certainly not an ordinary outcome of mature age, individuals must encounter some slight memory loss as they become more stated. The formation of plaques and tangles, abnormalities that could ultimately lead to dementia, can harm cells in the cerebrum and nerves.

4. The Stomach: A structure associated with your stomach. As you age, it turns out that your stomach-related is all the more firm and inflexible and does not contract as often. For example, stomach torment, obstruction, and feelings of nausea can prompt problems with this change; a superior diet can help.

5. The Abilities: You can see that your hearing and vision is not as good as it ever was. Maybe you'll start losing your sense of taste. Flavors might not appear as unique to you. Your odor and expertise in touch can also weaken. In order to respond, the body requires more time and needs more to revitalize it.

6. The Teeth: Throughout the years, the intense veneer protecting your teeth from rot will begin to erode, making you exposed to pits. Likewise, gum injury is a problem for more developed adults. Your teeth and gums will guarantee great dental cleanliness. Dry mouth, which is a common symptom of seniors' multiple drugs, can also be a concern.

7. The Skin: Your skin loses its versatility at a mature age and can tend to droop and wrinkle. Nonetheless, the more you covered your skin when you were younger from sun exposure and smoke, the healthier your skin would look as you get more mature. Start securing your skin right now to prevent more injury, much like skin malignancy.

8. The Sexual Conviviality: When the monthly period ends following menopause, many women undergo physical changes such as vaginal oil loss. Men can endure erectile brokenness. Fortunately, it is possible to handle the two problems successfully.

A normal part of maturing is a series of substantial improvements, but they don't need to back you up. Furthermore, you should do a lot to protect your body and keep it as stable as you would imagine, given the circumstances.

2.2. Keys to Aging Well

Although good maturation must preserve your physical fitness, it is also vital to appreciate the maturity and growth you acquire with propelling years. Its fine to rehearse healthy propensities for an extraordinary period, but it's never beyond the point of no return to gain the benefits of taking great account of yourself, even as you get more developed.

Here are some healthy maturing tips at every point of life that are a word of wisdom:

- Keep dynamic physically with a normal workout.

- With loved ones and inside your locale, remain socially diverse.

- Eat a balanced, well-adjusted diet, dumping low-quality food to intake low-fat, fiber-rich, and low-cholesterol.

- Do not forget yourself: daily enrollment at this stage with your primary care provider, dental surgeon, and optometrist is becoming increasingly relevant.

- Taking all medications as the primary care provider coordinates.

- Limit the consumption of liquor and break off smoke.

- Receive the rest your body wants.

Finally, it is necessary to deal with your physical self for a long time, but it is vital that you still have an eye on your passionate health. Receive and enjoy the rewards of your long life every single day. It is the perfect chance to enjoy better health and pleasure.

1. Eat a healthy diet

For more developed development, excellent nourishment and sanitation are especially critical. You need to regularly ensure that you eat a balanced, tailored diet. To help you decide on astute diet options and practice healthy nutrition, follow these guidelines.

2. Stay away from common medication mistakes

Drugs can cure health conditions and allow you to continue to lead a long, stable life. Drugs may also cause real health problems at the stage that they are misused. To help you decide on keen decisions about the remedy and over-the-counter medications you take, use these assets.

3. Oversee health conditions

Working with your healthcare provider to monitor health issues such as diabetes, osteoporosis, and hypertension is important. To treat these regular health problems, you need to get familiar with the medications and gadgets used.

4. Get screened

Health scans are an effective means of helping to perceive health conditions - even before any signs or side effects are given. Tell the healthcare provider what direct health scans are for you to determine how much you can be screened.

5. Be active

Exercise, as well as physical action, can help you to remain solid and fit. You just don't have to go to an exercise center. Converse about proper ways that you really can be dynamic with your healthcare professional. Look at the assets of the FDA and our accomplices in the administration.

2.3. Skin Sagging

There are also ways to prevent age from sagging, which are:

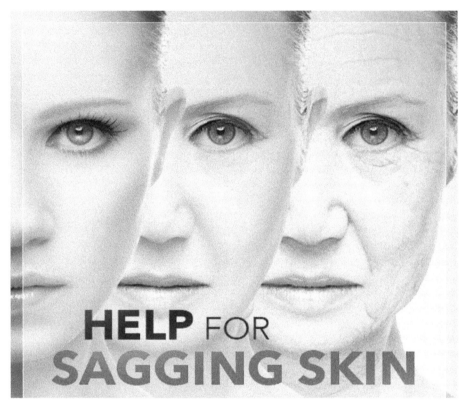

HELP FOR SAGGING SKIN

1. Unassuming Fixing and Lifting

These systems are called non-obtrusive methodologies of non-intrusive skin fixing on the basis that they leave your skin unblemished. A while later, you won't have a cut injury, a cut, or crude skin. You may see and grow some impermanent redness, but that is usually the main sign that you have a technique.

It is what you can expect from a skin-fixing method that is non-intrusive:

- **Results:** seem to come step by step, so they seem normal to be
- **Downtime:** zero to little
- **Colorblind:** secure for people with all skin hues
- **Body-wide use:** you can patch the skin almost anywhere on your body.

Ultrasonic dermatologists use ultrasound to transmit heat deep into the tissue.

Key concern: warming will induce more collagen to be created by your body. Many individuals see the unobtrusive raising and fixing within two and a half years of one procedure. By getting additional drugs, you can get more benefits.

During this procedure, the dermatologist places a radiofrequency device on the skin that warms the tissue beneath.

Key concern: Most people get one treatment and instantly feel an obsession. Your body needs some money to manufacture collagen, so you'll see the best effects in about half a year. By getting more than one treatment, a few persons benefit.

Some lasers will send heat deeply through the skin without injuring the skin's top layer by laser therapy. These lasers are used to repair skin everywhere and can be especially effective for fixing free skin on the tummy and upper arms.

Primary concern: to get outcomes, you may need 3 to 5 drugs, which occur step by step somewhere in the region of 2 and a half years after the last procedure.

2. Most fixing and lifting without medical procedure

While these methodologies will deliver you increasingly measurable results, considering all, they will not give you the aftereffects of an operation such as a facelift, eyelid surgical treatment, or neck lift, insignificantly pleasing to the eye skin fixing techniques. Negligibly obtrusive skin fixing requires less personal time than surgical treatment, however. It also conveys less chance of reactions.

3. How to look younger than your age without Botox, lasers and surgery, plus natural remedies for skin sagging

It is possible to become more experienced in this lifetime. However, you don't need to look at your age on the off chance you'd like not to. Truth be told, if you have been wondering how you would look as youthful as you feel, we will be eager to bet that you feel a lot more youthful than the amount you call your "age!"

2.4. Weight loss

Quality preparation builds the quality of your muscles and improves your versatility.

Even though cardio is very important for lung health and the heart, getting more fit and keeping it off is anything but an incredible technique.

The weight will return quickly at the point when you quit doing a lot of cardio. An unquestionable requirement has cardio as a component of your general wellness routine; be that as it may, when you start going to the exercise centre, quality preparation should be the primary factor. Quality preparation increases your muscle's quality, but this will enhance your portability and the main thing known to build bone thickness (alongside appropriate supplements).

Weight-bearing exercises help build and maintain bulk and build bone quality and reduce the risk of osteoporosis. Many people over [the age of] 50 will stop regularly practicing due to torment in their joints or back or damage, but do not surrender. In any case, understand that because of age-related illness, hormone changes, and even social variables such as a busy life, it may seem more enthusiastic to pick up muscle as you age. As he would like to think that to build durable muscles, cardio will consume off fat and pick substantial weights with few representatives or lighter weights. Similarly, for generally speaking health and quality, remember exercise and diet are linked to the hip, likewise, as the trick of the year. ! Locate a professional who can help you get back into the groove and expect to get 2 hrs.

Thirty minutes of physical movement in any case [in] seven days to help to maintain your bulk and weight.

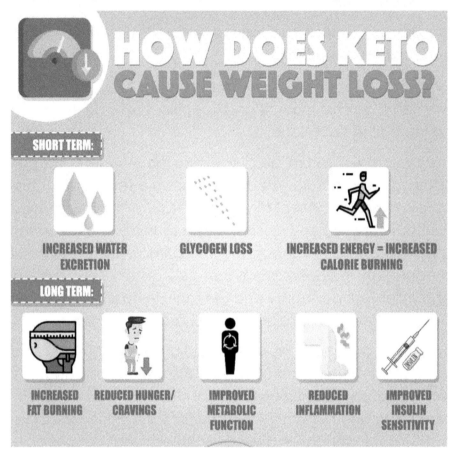

1. Try not to skip meals.

Testosterone and Estrogen decline gradually after some time, which also prompts fat collection because the body does not prepare sugar. We alternatively keep losing more bulk as we get older; this will cause our bodies' metabolic needs to lessen. Be that as it may, meal skipping can make you lack significant key medications required as we age, for example, by before large protein and calories. Tracking your energy levels throughout the day and obtaining sufficient calories/protein would also help you feel better on the scale, explaining how you will be burning more calories but less inefficiently. We also lose more bulk as we age, causing our metabolic rate to decrease. Be that as it may, skipping meals can make you lack important key supplements required as we age, for example, by an aging, metabolic rate.

2. Ensure you are getting enough rest.

"Perhaps the highest argument of over 50 years is a lack of rest," Amselem notes. Basically, rest may interfere with an important medical procedure, causing metabolic breakage in the system, in which the body turns weakness into hunger, urging you to eat. I plan to rest for seven to eight hours and, if necessary, take low rest. Rest is vital to a healthy weight because two hormones, leptin, and Ghrelin are released during rest, and they conclude a significant job in eating guidelines.

3. Relinquish old "rules" about weight loss and develop an outlook on health.

For the two women and men, age impacts weight loss, and that is on the basis that digestion backs off, hormone levels decay, in addition to there is a loss of bulk," "Nevertheless, that does not imply that mission is inconceivable to get more fit over age 50. Everybody else has to take a half hour's exercise, but there are two big reasons why it can't be done: you eat too much, or you are not active enough. The wellness movement encourages people to be aware of their own health, body and well-being. Being over 50 years old is not the end of the world. In fact, there is still a chance for us to live the rest of our lives as retirees. It is important to eat well, exercise, not smoke, and limit alcohol consumption in our lives. Our bodies are naturally aging, but we do not yet have to quit. Instead of falling prey to craze diets, make ongoing acclimatization to advance adjusted eating, and help yourself remember the benefits of exercise for your heart, stomach-related tract, and psychological well-being, despite the executives' weight.

2.5. Factors Influencing Fuel Utilization

The amount of each element in one's blood plasma determines the combination of fuels in the body. According to the researchers, the main element that determines how much of each nutrient is absorbed is the quantity of each nutrient eaten first by the body. The second considerations to take into account when assessing one's health is the amounts of hormones like insulin and glucagon, which must be in balance with one's diet. The third is the body's physical accumulation (cellular) of any nutrient, such as fat, muscle, and liver glycogen. Finally, the quantities of regulatory enzymes for glucose & fat breakdown beyond our influence, but changes in diet and exercise decide each gasoline's overall usage. Surely, both of these considerations will be discussed more extensively below.

1. Quantity of nutrients consumed

Humans will obtain four calories from sources in their surroundings: carbon, hydrogen, nitrogen, and oxygen. When it comes to the body demanding and using a given energy supply, it prefers to choose the nearest one to it due to the quantity and concentration in the bloodstream. The body can improve its use of glucose or decrease its use of glucose directly due to the amount of carbohydrate intake being ingested. It is an effort by the liver to control glycogen (sugar) levels in the body. If carbohydrate (carb) intake goes up, the use of carbohydrate-containing goods will go up, in exchange. Proteins are slightly harder to control. As protein consumption goes up, our bodies increase their development and oxidation of proteins as well. The food source for our body is protein. If it is in short supply, our body will consume less of it. This is an attempt to keep body protein cellular levels stable at 24-hour intervals. Since dietary fat does not lift the amount of fat the body needs, it cannot dramatically change how much fuel the body gets from that fat. Rather than measuring insulin directly, it is important to measure insulin indirectly, so it does not drift.

The blood alcohol content can decrease the body's energy reserves with those calories of fat. This will almost entirely impair the body's usage of fat for food. As most people know, carbohydrate intake will influence the amount of fat the body uses as a fuel supply. High carb diets increase the body's use of fat for food and the insulin threshold and amount. Therefore, the highest fat oxidation rates occur when there are low levels of carbohydrates in the body. Another clarification of this can be found in chapter 18, where it is clarified that the amount of glycogen regulates how much fat is used by the muscles. When a human eats less energy and carbohydrates, the body can subsequently take up fat calories for food instead of carbohydrates.

2. Hormone levels

Factors like food, exercise, medications and hormones all play a part in how we use our bodies' fuel. The hormone known as insulin is of high interest to many physicians because it plays a significant role in a wide range of activities, including the bodies functioning. A glance at the hormones involved in fuel consumption is included in the following passage.

Insulin is a peptide (as in the "peptide" in "peptides" that are essential in digestion) that the pancreas releases in response to changes in blood glucose. As blood glucose goes up, insulin levels also rise, and the body will use this extra glucose to kind of store it as glycogen in the muscles or in the liver. Glucose and extra glucose will be forced into fat cells for preservation (as alpha-glycerophosphate). Protein synthesis is enhanced, and as a result, amino acids (the building blocks of proteins) are transferred out of the blood via muscle cells and are then placed together to make bigger proteins. Fat synthesis or "lipogenesis" (making fat) and fat accumulation are also induced. In effect, it's hard for insulin to be released from fat cells due to even tiny levels of it. The main objective of insulin is regulating blood glucose in a very small range of around 80 to 120 milligrams per decilitre. When blood glucose levels rise outside of the normal range, insulin is released to get the glucose levels back into a normal range. The greatest rise in blood glucose levels (and the greatest increase in insulin) happens when humans eat carbohydrates in the diet. Due to amino acids that can be converted to glycogen, the breakdown of proteins can cause an increase the amount of insulin released. FFA can induce insulin release and produce ketone bodies found at concentrations that are far smaller than those produced by carbohydrates or proteins.

When your glucose level decreases, as it does with exercise and from eating less carbohydrate, your insulin levels decrease as well. During cycles with low insulin and higher hormones, the body's storage fuels can burst, leading to a breakdown of stored fuels. After accumulation within the body, triglycerides are broken down into fatty acids and glycerol and released into the bloodstream. Specific proteins might be broken down into individual amino acids and used as sources of sources glucose. Glycogen is a material contained in the liver that is broken when insulin is absent. Failure to produce insulin suggests a pathological state. Type me, diabetes (or Insulin Dependent Diabetes Mellitus, IDDM). In a group of patients with Type I diabetes (1), these patients have a deficiency in the pancreas, causing them to be entire without insulin. I already told you that to practical control glucose levels, people with diabetes have to inject themselves with insulin. This is relevant in the next chapter since the difference between diabetic ketoacidosis and dietary mediated ketosis is made in the chapter after this. Glucagon is essentially known as insulin's mirror hormone in the body and has nearly opposite effects. The enzyme insulin is also a peptide hormone made by the pancreas, which is released from the cells of the body, and its primary function as well is to sustain stable glucose levels. However, once blood glucose goes down below average, glucagon increases blood glucose on its own. The precursors are expelled from the cells into the bloodstream.

Glucagon's key function is in the liver, where it signals the degradation of liver glycogen and the resulting release into the bloodstream. The release of glucagon is modulated by what we eat, the sort of workout, and the presence of a meal that activates the development of glucagon in the body (24). High amounts of insulin suppress the pancreas from releasing the hormone glucagon. Normally, glucagon's actions are restricted to the liver; by comparison, its function in these other tissues is yet to be detected (i.e., fat and muscle cells). On the other hand, when insulin levels are very low, such as when glucose restriction and activity occur, glucagon plays a minor role in fat mobilization, as well as the degradation of muscle glycogen. Glucagon's primary function is to regulate blood glucose under conditions of low blood sugar. But it also plays a crucial role in ketone body development in the liver, which we will address in-depth in the next chapter. Below are the definitions of two contrasting hormones. It should be obvious from reading the sentences that they have opposite effects on one another. Whereas insulin is a key storage hormone that allows for the retention of accumulated glucose, potassium, albumin and fat in the body, glucagon serves the same role by allowing for the utilization of stored fat in an organism.

Insulin and glucagon are central to the determination to be anabolic or catabolic. However, their presence in the body is not alone enough for muscle development. Other hormones are involved as well. They will briefly be discussed below. Growth hormone, which is a peptide hormone, elicits various effects on the body, such as its effects on blood flow and muscle tissue growth. The hormone to hold appetite at bay, Ghrelin, is released in response to several stressors. Most notably, exercise, a reduction in blood glucose, and carbohydrate restriction or fasting can both induce Ghrelin production. As its name suggests (GH), GH is a growth-promoting hormone, which enhances protein production (protein synthesis) in the body and liver. Glucose, glycogen, and triglycerides also are mobilized from fat cells for nutrition.

Adrenaline and noradrenaline (also called epinephrine and norepinephrine) are members of a special family of hormones called 'fight or flight' hormones. They tend to be released in response to discomfort, such as running, fasting, or consuming cold foods. Epinephrine is a drug that is emitted from the adrenal medulla, passing across the bloodstream to the brain to exert its effects on several tissues of the body. The impacts of the catecholamine's on the different tissues of the body are very involved and maybe the subject of a research paper. The primary function of catecholamine metabolites affecting the ketogenic diet was to increase fatty acids excretion in the urine and increase fatty acids in the blood. When it's hard for someone to change their ways, it's because their insulin levels aren't where they should be. The only hormone that actually affects fat mobilization is insulin. Like the Catecholamine's, insulin and insulin mimics have a corresponding effect on fat mobilization.

3. Liver glycogen

The liver is one of the most metabolically active organs in the whole human body. Although everything we consume is not digested immediately by the stomach, this is part of the whole digestion process. Like the body, the degree to which the liver retains glycogen is the dominating influence to the extent to which the body will retain or break down nutrients. It is typically (hesitation) because there is a higher body fat level associated with elevated liver glycogen levels. The liver is analogous to a short term stead storehouse and glycogen source regulating blood glucose in our body. After the liver releases more glucose into the blood, more glucagon is released, which activates the breaking down of liver glycogen to glucose, to be introduced into the bloodstream. When the liver has glycogen stocks completely, blood glucose levels are retained, and the body enters the anabolic state, meaning the incoming glucose, amino acids, and free fatty acids are all processed as these three molecules, respectively. This is often referred to as 'the fed establishment.' Red blood cells can't hold as much oxygen as they did when filled with massive amounts of glycogen, so they release it when they're no longer needed and transform into the liver. The body cuts edible protein into amino acids, which are then placed into the formation of amino acids, and finally, will produce for you fats and sugars. This is often referred to as the 'fasted' condition.

4. Enzyme levels

Precise control of fuel consumption in the body is done through the action of enzymes. Ultimately, enzyme levels are calculated by the carbohydrates that are being consumed in the diet and the hormone levels which are caused by it. On the other hand, where there is a surplus of carbohydrates in one's diet, this form of dietary shift stimulates insulin's influence on the cells' ability to utilize glucose and prevent fatty stores' degradation. Thus, if there is a decrease in insulin levels, the enzymes are blocked, which results in a drop in the enzymes involved in glucose usage and in fats breakdown. A long term adjustment to a high carbohydrate / low carbohydrate diet may induce longer-term modifications in the enzymes involved in fats and carbohydrates, resulting in long term changes in the core. If you limit carbohydrate consumption for many weeks, this will deplete enzymes' liver and muscle and transfer them to be brought upon the liver and muscle that concerns fat burning. The result of disrupting the balance of dietary components is an inability to use carbs for fuel for some time after food is reintroduced to the diet.

Chapter 3: Keto with Intermittent Fasting

This chapter will give you a detailed view to the Keto with intermittent fasting.

Intermittent fasting, in a more condensed definition, allows people to miss a meal daily. The popular forms of intermittent fasting include the one day fast, a 24 hour fast or a 5:2 fast, where people eat very little food for a predetermined number of days, then consume lots of food (ADF). The intermittent fasting function of IF breaks the subjects fasting routine every other day. Unlike crash diets that frequently produce rapid results but can be hard to sustain for the long run, both intermittent fasting and keto Diet focus on the real root systems of how the body absorbs food and how you make your dietary decisions for each day. Intermittent eating and Keto diets should be practiced as dietary modification. They are long-term options for a better, happier you.

It is where the biggest distinction lies among IF and Interval feeding (TRF). The TRF is the fast of restricting the feeding time to between 4-10 hours during the day and missing the fasting time the rest of the time. All or most people who observe intermittent fasting do so regularly.

3.1. What Is Ketosis?

From the outside looking in, carbs appear to be a simple and fast means of bringing nutrients right through the day. Think of all those grab-and-go and protein-filled snacks that we equate with breakfast—granola bars, fruit-filled muffins, smoothies. We start our mornings by eating many carbs, and then later on in the day, they add more carbs. Just because a given technology works does not make it the most effective way. To keep us safe, the tissues and cells that produce our bodies require energy to fulfil their daily functions. There are two main sources of strength in the foods we consume, but the first source is non-animal, and the second source is animal. One source of energy is the carbohydrate, which transforms into glucose. At this time, this is the process that most people go through. These cars have an alternative fuel, however, and a shocking one: fat. No, the very thing any doctor has recommended you to reduce your lifelong lifespan may be the weapon you need to jump-start your metabolism. During this process, tiny organic molecules, called Ketone, are emitted from our body, signalling that the food we eat is being broken down. Ketones are actual nutrients that help run much of our body's cells, including muscles. You've undoubtedly heard the term "Metabolism" repeated in one's life, but do you understand what it means exactly as a fast-acting chemical process? In short, this is alkaline, causing effective cellular functioning, which can be present in any type of living thing. Considering that humans are extremely difficult in many ways, our bodies generally process simpler things like food and exercise. Our bodies are actively struggling to do their jobs. And whether we are either asleep or not, our cells are actively constructing and restoring. The robots ought to remove the energetic particles from inside our bodies.

Around the same time, glucose, which is what carbohydrates are broken down into after we ingest them, is a critical component in the process of bringing sugar into the body. We are now concentrating our diet on carbs as the main source of calories for our body. Without mentioning the fructose we eat as well as the recommended daily servings of fruit, starchy veggies, and starchy vegetables, as well as plant-based sources of protein, there is no shortage of glucose in our bodies. The problem with this type of energy use is that this results in us buying into the recycling-focused consumerism that is a by-product of the half-baked technologies. Our bodies get hammered by the number of calories we eat every day. Some people are eating more than they need, and that can contribute to obesity.

Most people cannot reach ketosis quickly, but you can reach it by exercising, eating less, and drinking a decent amount of water. As was seen through the data, our current "Food Pyramid," which instructs us to consume a high amount of carbohydrate-rich foods as energy sources, is turned upside down. A more effective formula for feeding your body has fats at the top, making up 60 to 80 percent of your diet; protein in the middle at 20 to 30 percent; and carbs (real glucose in disguise) way at the bottom, accounting for only 5 to 10 percent of your regular eating plan.

3.2. Paleo vs. Keto

Evolution has many opportunities to bring. We can use fire and energy to cook our food is evidence enough that change can be a positive thing about our lives. Anywhere between our trapper foraging lifestyle and the industrialized lifestyle we have today, there is a significant disconnect. Although our lifespans have improved, we're not winning from the longevity of those additional years because our health is being undermined. The tired, unclear sensation you are having might be not just because you need to get more sleep - it may be because you lack vitamin B12 in your diet. If we eat food as fuel for our bodies, it's fair to assume that what we eat has a big effect on our productivity. If you burn fuel in an engine designed to run on gasoline, there could be some very harmful consequences. Is it conceivable that our bodies have set up this insulin receptor cascade to only accept sugar, in a process comparable to our transition to providing fat as a rapid source of energy rather than a source of energy for our early ancestors? I know this sounds an awful lot like arguing for a Paleo diet, but although the ketogenic lifestyle seems similar, keto's basic concept is vastly different. Ketosis happens when you eat fewer calories and change the intake of protein and fat. There are many medicinal effects of ketosis, and the primary one is quick weight loss (fat, protein, carbohydrates, fiber, and fluids). Per calorie is made up of four distinct types of macronutrients. Many considerations go into the certain food decisions that a person makes, and it's crucial to consider one's emotions.

Fiber makes us regular, for instance, and it lets food flows into the digestive tract. What goes in has to come out, and for that process, fiber is necessary. Protein helps to heal tissue, generate enzymes and to create bones, muscles and skin. Liquids keep us hydrated; our cells, muscles, and organs do not operate correctly without them. The primary function of carbohydrates is to supply energy, but the body must turn them into glucose to do so, which has a ripple effect on the body's parts. Because of its link to insulin production through higher blood sugar levels, a carb intake is a balancing act for persons with diabetes. Good fats stimulate cell formation, protect our lungs, help keep us warm, and supply nutrition, but only in small amounts when carbs are ingested. I'm going to explain more about when and how this is happening soon.

3.3. Carbs vs. Net Carbs

In virtually any food supply, carbohydrates occur in some type. Total carbohydrate reduction is unlikely and unrealistic. To work, we want some carbohydrates. If we want to learn that certain foods that drop into the restricted group on a keto diet become better options than others, it's important to understand this.

In the caloric breakdown of a meal, fiber counts as a carb. It is interesting to remember is that our blood sugar is not greatly impaired by fiber, a positive thing because it is an integral macronutrient that allows us better digest food. You're left with what's considered net carbs after subtracting the sum of fiber from the number of carbs in the caloric tally of an element or finished recipe. Think of your pay check before (gross) taxes and after (net). A bad comparison, maybe, because no one wants to pay taxes, but an efficient one to try to explain and track carbs versus net carbs. You place a certain amount of carbohydrates in your bloodstream, but any of them does not influence your blood sugar content.

It doesn't mean that with whole-grain pasta, you may go mad. Although it's a better alternative than flour of white-coloured pasta, you can limit your net carbs to 20 - 30 grams per day total. To place that in context, approximately 35 g of carbohydrates and just 7 grams of total fiber are found in two ounces of undercooked whole-grain pasta. Pasta and bread are undoubtedly the two key things people would ask you if you miss them.

3.4. When does ketosis kick in?

Most individuals go through ketosis within a few days. People who are different will take a week to adapt. Factors that cause ketosis include existing body mass, diet, and exercise levels. Ketosis is a moderate state of ketosis since ketone levels would be low for a longer time. One can calculate ketone levels in a structured way, but you can note certain biological reactions that indicate you are in ketosis. There are not as serious or drastic symptoms, and benefits can outweigh risks in this phase-in time, so it is good to be familiar with symptoms in case they arise.

Starvation vs. Fasting

Make a deliberate decision to fast. The biggest differentiator between going on a fast and feeding intermittently is that it is your choice to continue fasting. The amount of time you want to fast and the reason for fasting are not imposed upon you by the hospital, whether it is for religious practices, weight loss, or a prolonged detox cycle. Most fasting is performed at will. When fasting, proper feeding has clear implications on the overall way of our well-being. A series of situations can bring about starvation out of the hands of the people suffering from those conditions. Starvation, hunger, and war are but a couple of these conditions to be caused by a devastated economy. Starvation is starvation due to lack of the proper nutrients that can lead to organ failure and ultimately death. No one wants to live without calories.

When I knew that avoiding smoking would help my health, I immediately wondered, "Why do I continue to smoke?"

And once I learn about the motivations for doing this, it is much easier to see them. I have also been concerned about the early days of fasting. Before I knew that there is a distinction between fasting and starvation and that it is safe, my first response to the thought of not eating and starving was still, "Why would anyone choose to kill themselves with starving?." As for this article's intent, someone who fasts is just opting not to eat for a predetermined amount of time. Even nonviolent vigils that are meant to oppose using a certain form of killing feed larger and larger gatherings.

Would your hunger vanish before the fast?

So that's a brilliant query; let's try a couple more angles. The fact is, we all eat a full meal once a day. It is a normal tradition that we eat our last meal a few hours before going to sleep, and all but breastfeeding new-borns do not eat the moment they wake up. And if you devote just a limit of six hours a night to sleep, you are likely to be fasting ten hours a day anyway. Now, let's begin to incorporate the concept in periodic to the formula. Anything that is "intermittent" implies something that is not constant. When adding it to the concept of fasting, it means you're lengthening the time that you don't eat between meals (the term "breakfast" means only that, breaking the fast).

From fasting once a day, we have an established "mind over matter" power. What will be a major concern, though, would be mind over mind. We will come back to the issue of how you feel after you stop feeding. The first week of fasting may change as you get used to the prolonged amount of time of your current intermittent fasting target. All of the fasting periods that I have given allow you timewise to adapt to the Ketogenic Diet and this method adjusts your sleeping routine so that it suits them. It is conceivable (and likely) that your body will start to feel hungry about 10 a.m., around the moment it usually eats lunch. But, after one day, you can adapt, and after a couple of days, you should no longer have trouble feeding before noon.

To support you before making the shift you're playing with, observe what happens when you put back the first meal of the day by an extra thirty minutes per day for a week. This way, as you begin the schedule set out here, you'll need to change the timing of your final meal of the day just after you begin week two of the plan for the Meals from Noon to 6 p.m. No appointments are required.

3.5. Why Prefer Intermittent Fasting?

Now that you have learned that it is possible to fast without starving to death and that it is also a deliberate decision, you might think, why on earth you would ever choose to fast. Its ability to encourage weight loss is one of the key reasons that IF has taken the diet world by storm. Metabolism is one feature of the human body. Metabolism requires two basic reactions: catabolism and anabolism.

Catabolism is the portion of metabolism where our bodies break down food. Catabolism involves breaking down large compounds into smaller units. The body uses the energy from the food we consume to produce new cells, build muscles, and sustain organs. This term is often referred to as parallel or dual catabolism and anabolism. A diet routine that sees us eating most of the day means our bodies have less time to waste in the anabolic process of metabolism. It is hard to find out since they are related, but note that they occur at different rates. The most significant point is that a prolonged fasting time allows for optimum metabolic efficiency.

The improved mental acuity has an intrinsic influence of improving attention, focus, concentration and focus. According to various reports, fasting made you more alert and concentrated, not sleepy or light-headed. Many people point to nature and our desire to survive. We may not have had food preservation, but we lived day to day, regardless of how ample food supplies may have been.

Scientists agree that fasting often heightens neurogenesis, the growth and regeneration of nerve tissue in the brain. Both paths lead to the fact that fasting gives the body enough time to do routine maintenance. You extend the time you give your body to concentrate on cellular growth and tissue recovery by sleeping longer between your last meal and your first meal.

Are Fluids Allowed While Fasting?

The last important detail for intermittent fasting is that it speeds up the metabolism; unlike religious fasting, which also forbids food consumption during the fast period, an IF requires you to drink a certain liquid during the fast time. You are not consuming something that is caloric; therefore, this action breaks the fast. As we can glean from its strong weight loss record, a closer look through the prism of intermittent fasting can yield very promising outcomes. Bone broth (here) is the beneficiary of both the nutrients and vitamins and can refill the sodium amounts. Permission has been given to use coffee and tea without any sweeteners and ideally without any milk or cream. There are two separate schools of thinking about applying milk or soda to your coffee or tea. Provided it's just a high-fat addition, such as coconut oil or butter to make bulletproof coffee (here), many keto supporters believe it's a waste of time and not properly gain sufficient protein. Using MCT oil, it is assumed that people can obtain more energy and be happier moving on with their daily lives. Coffee and tea drinkers tend toward simple brews. It is perfect for you to choose whichever strategy you want, as long as you don't end up "alternating" between the two techniques. I often recommend drinking water, as staying hydrated is necessary for any healthier choice a person can make. Caffeine use can be very depleting, so be careful to control your water intake and keep yourself balanced.

Conclusions:

An important element to note is eating a great combination of lean meat, greens, and unprocessed carbs. The most efficient way to eat a balanced diet is simply adhering to whole foods, mainly because it is a healthy solution. It is crucial to understand that it is impossible to complete a ketogenic diet.

If you're a woman over 50, you may be far more interested in weight loss. Many women experience decreased metabolism at this age at a rate of about 50 calories per day. It can be incredibly hard to control weight gain by slowing the metabolism combined with less activity, muscle degradation and the potential for greater cravings. Many food options can help women over 50 lose weight and maintain healthy habits, but the keto diet has recently been one of the most popular.

Lightning Source UK Ltd.
Milton Keynes UK
UKHW010634250621
386141UK00010B/353

9 781802 268928